I0408995

NCD
Flaxseed Shake
recipe™

taken from the first 46 pages of

12 Changes a Year

Volume 1

the recipe book to the

Number Crunch Diet

Jumper Publications and Media

Disclaimer

The purpose of this book is to empower the reader with knowledge, to educate, informational purposes. This book is not medical advice, but rather the author's personal experience, and is a guide for anyone who wishes to implement said dietary or lifestyle changes at the reader's own discretion. The choice between medical care and self care is completely up to the reader. If you have a medical problem, seek medical care. The author and Jumper Publications and Media shall not be held responsible or liable for any and all damages, loss, or injury, of any kind that may be caused or allegedly caused, directly or indirectly, by the information in this book. Reading beyond this page is the reader's consent to the above disclaimer.

Other Publications

ABC Water and the Number Crunch Diet
a step by step solution to alkaline deficiency and
with a New and Unique approach to weight control

Nontoxic Teeth Whitening and Dental Hygiene System
"Spare me the chemicals, I've switched to FOOD GRADE to
whiten, gargle and brush."

JPM Oral Hygiene Protocol
stop using toxic drugstore mouthwash, discover how to reduce
your gum pocket depth from 3-4-3 to 1-2-1 mm when they probe

12 Changes A Year – Volume 1
the recipe book to the Number Crunch Diet
When you take control of the numbers
you take control of your weight.

The 5 Points of Posture
the missing link to fat loss, overall wellness, and
to becoming Respected, Adored, and Wealthy

12 Changes A Year – Volume 2
the recipe book to the Number Crunch Diet
Begin today and forever be in control of the numbers you're eating.

Vision Is Possible
Improve your vision and get a facelift for free!
an original vision program targeting your Eye Lids

To purchase additional copies, please visit

http://www.CreateSpace.com/4910129

CONTENTS

1	NCD Flaxseed Shake™	1
2	NCD Omega 3 Protocol™	6
3	Milk & Ellen White	12
4	NCD Mineral Shake™	19
5	NCD Secret Ingredient™	25
6	KEY PROTEIN	31
7	The Numbers!	35
8	NCD FSR Variations™	41
	Preview	47
	TCY – 2	48
	Free Report – JPM Oral Hygiene Protocol™ #1	49
	Free Report – JPM Oral Hygiene Protocol™ #2	55
	Follow-up	61
	Top Ten	62
	Quiz	64

Edits & Format

You will notice oddities in punctuation, spelling, syntax, and perhaps even semantics, within this book. Feel free to let me know, but some of it is done for brevity or to shift emphasis. I use capitals where I see fit, to grab your attention and make it stand out, and I also remove capitals when I don't think they are deserving of them, or to remove emphasis after first usage, i.e., Pyrex becomes pyrex. And french bread, brussels sprouts, and english cucumbers, are spelled lowercase, as we are not going to "link" a European vacation to our food and eating.

Secondly, I will unhyphenate to create rhythm. Grammatically, two or more words that function as an adjective before a noun are supposed to be hyphenated. That's fine. A million-dollar smile, is the adjective "million-dollar" describing the smile. However, this can get redundant after a while, 1&2 3, 1&2 3, 1&2 3. The noun gets all the attention. But what if you want the adjectives to have the emphasis? After all, the adjectives are the descriptive words. So, I will drop the hyphens to allow the adjectives equal emphasis, and to change the pace of the sentence a bit. So if there are no hyphens, read it slower and evenly, one two three four five six seven. A "step-by-step solution" sounds a bit skippy and simplistic, whereas, a "step by step solution" is said slower and sounds more methodical. Hyphenating two words, or joining two words as a compound word, reduces their individual meanings.

With regard to fastfood, healthfood, and seasalt, it's time for these words to evolve into compound words, so the trend starts here.

There are also some fragmented sentences, subject-verb disagreements, and singular/plural violations. When "correcting" certain of these sentences, they lost their emphasis and punch, so I kept them as is.

In the past I've been guilty of judging other author's sentences, only to reread it with the commas, pauses, and then it made perfect sense. So, if there's a comma, then pause, as you may not get to pause later in the sentence. If there's no comma, then don't pause and read it all as one.

I pose questions, but without question marks. Some are rhetorical, but some are to make you Ponder. Great word. Ponder. If you see a question mark at the end, then it requires an answer. If there's no question mark, then you can just say, yeah, no, or hm.

English continues to change, people using it, customize the language to fit what they want to communicate, emphasize, and to make their point from various angles. It also has to have a variety of melodies and rhythms to keep it from being boring. If you find yourself having to reread a sentence, it may be that it's structured that way for that very reason. So take your time. Don't rush. Let the words digest, so that you absorb the material, and hopefully take some of it and make it a part of your life.

Lastly, you will notice that I customized the headers of every page! This is not something Microsoft Word Starter allows you to do. You can only customize three pages, first, even, and odd. So, to get around this I had to create a Page Break every three pages, and as a result, the last line of some of the pages doesn't "justify" to the edge. So I hope that flipping through the upper corners of the pages will assist you in finding the chapter that you are looking for.

You won't see any citations from scientific studies or PubMed, because at JPM we look to a higher source for our reference.

God Bless!

Enjoy the Journey

Email me if you have a question, or if you just want to comment. Your purchase comes with 6-months free support and photos.

Barry Ogston, B.Sc., CLS, MLS(ASCP)

You have to crunch the numbers to see what you're really eating.

CHAPTER 1

NCD FLAXSEED SHAKE™

Hi! Welcome Back!

Hopefully you've read *ABC Water and the Number Crunch Diet*. Assuming this to be the case, let me tell you how Awesome! I think you are, as getting good nutrition and maintaining weight through calorie control are, in my opinion, key answers to good health and longevity.

I wish we had a word in our vocabulary for "looking half your age". If you are 40 and look 20, or you're 60 and look 30-ish, this says it all. These people have health, longevity, energy, and this should really be the desired goal. You don't age. Or you don't age much. Not nearly as much as everyone else. You stand out. You're a freak of nature, defying space and time! I say, Go For It!

This chapter, I believe, is a tool in helping you to achieve this goal. The NCD Flaxseed Shake™ is the most amazing of my inventions. Why? Because flax seeds ground fresh and consumed fresh is the only safe guarantee that you will be consuming those unstable "U" shaped omega-3 fatty acids in their true "U" shaped form.

See, saturated fats, like butter and coconut oil, are relatively stable fats. Coconut oil, since it lacks dairy, can last up to two years at room temperature without spoiling. These saturated fatty acids are straight-line chains. No bends, no twists, no contortions.

In a cell membrane, these saturated straight-line fatty acids provide the cell with rigidity. This is good. But within that rigid ring membrane, we need some flexible points. This is where Omega-3 comes in.

The best way to get omega-3 is by grinding fresh organic flax seeds and consuming them right away, or, in my case, I grind two servings, have one now, and one within 24 hours, keeping the second serving in an airtight container in the refrigerator.

It's similar to an apple spoiling after you cut into it, or strawberries gradually going south in a couple of days. Flax seeds, once ground, need to be consumed right away.

The recipe requires four items.
1. organic flax seeds
2. raw whole milk
3. NCD Secret Protein™
4. blackstrap molasses
This is the NCD Molasses Flaxseed Shake™

There are two other versions. The NCD Maple Flaxseed Shake™, where you will substitute Grade B maple syrup for the molasses, and the NCD Honey Flaxseed Shake™, substituting Raw Unfiltered honey for the molasses.

1. Certified Organic Golden Flax Seeds
I purchase this from Bush Creek Organic Foods, on the web at www.bcof.com, (800) 630-5916. This is the best flaxseed at the best price. The label says, "Grown without chemicals, fungicides, herbicides, or pesticides, and involves no genetically modified organisms, GMOs." Then it says, "In order to get the most benefit from your whole flax seeds, grind them fresh and just before using." See, this company understands that omega-3 fat is unstable and spoils quickly once ground – smart people.

The current cost for 12 one-pound bags is $83.88 plus $16.04 UPS shipping, which averages out to $8.33 per bag, and they are still throwing in a free coffee grinder with the 12-bag purchase. Their website has a lot of information about the health benefits of flax seeds and the quality of their product. I am already a believer in flax, but if you still need convincing, I recommend you read their site. This is definitely a great group of farmers. Thank you Bush Creek!

There is only one ingredient, omega golden flax seeds, certified organic. Plus, this part of the country (North Dakota), is away from freeways and air pollution. Any time you can SEE the air, that's not good for crops.

Nutrition Facts
2T 20g
servings per container ~23 (the "~" sign means approximately)
E = 110 calories per 2 Tablespoons/20 grams
F = 70 calories from fat
total Fat = 8g x9 = 72cal (about the same as F=70)(fat x9=cals)
SF = 1g x9 = 9cal of saturated fat
Omega-3 = 3.8g x9 = 34.2cal
Omega-6 = 1.3g x9 = 11.7cal
Omega-9 = 1.8g x9 = 16.2cal
TF = 0 trans fat=0 per NCD rules
Chol = 0mg cholesterol is not found in plant food
Na = 0mg no sodium
K = 170mg some potassium
CHO = 5g x4 = 20 calories of carbohydrate (carb grams x4=cals)
f = 12g x4 = 48 calories of fiber
s = 0g no sugar
Prot = 4g x4 = 16 calories of protein (prot grams x4=cals)
T = 108 total calories

When we add up our three macros, fat carbs prot, 72 + 20 + 16, we get 108 calories, or T = 108. This is pretty close to the E = 110, but labels aren't perfect. The energy is listed in calories at the top, but you should always calculate it yourself by adding up the fat carbs protein. I call this T, total calories. Also notice the discrepancy in F, fat cals = 70 and our calculated fat cals of 72.

The fiber calories of 48 is higher than the total carb calories of 20, so you may ask, how can this be? I called them and they said that the government makes the Nutrition Facts, they just send the product in for analysis. This leads us to the whole debate about whether you CAN subtract the fiber calories from the carb number. Brace yourselves, as I'll do the best I can.

Insoluble fiber doesn't get absorbed, it stays within the colon, adding bulk to your stool, so it has no calories. Soluble fiber gets absorbed into the body, so it has calories, but it creates a gel gelatin like material that slows down the glycemic load of your meal.

In the USA, the FDA says that companies can subtract the insoluble-fiber grams from the total-carb grams. In Canada, food companies cannot. So, if you buy food in the United States, the manufacturer has likely already subtracted the insoluble fiber from the carbs so you don't want to do it again when you crunch your numbers.

However, there is no consistency and no indication that food companies are doing this and if so which ones are and which ones aren't. This is the gray area of the food label, and so we have to rely on our body's signals and intuition.

If you feel "low energy" after a meal, chances are there weren't enough sugar carbs, or, the soluble gel fiber is slowing down the release of sugar too much. Therefore, you will want to increase the carbs slightly by 3-4% to 43 or 44%. This way, when you subtract the fiber carbs, you end up with closer to 40% carbs.

If the meal leaves you feeling a bit bloated, that "fat gain" feeling, your meal may have too many sugar carbs and the glycemic load is a bit high. In this situation, you will NOT subtract the fiber carbs from your total carbs.

You can also eat the meal slower if you find it has high sugar and it's making you feel fat after eating it. The NCD Shakes have some sugar. Maple syrup, molasses, and honey are powerful sugars. But they are also healthy sugars. This brings us to the:

NCD Five Healthy Sugars™
1. Molasses – blackstrap
2. Maple Syrup – grade B
3. Honey – raw, unfiltered
4. Fruit
5. Cane Sugar – organic, minimally refined

Molasses is unrefined syrup from sugarcane or sugar beets.
Grade B maple syrup, tree sap, is less refined than grade A.
Honey, raw unfiltered, is unrefined sugar from a beehive.
Fruit, fresh in-season fruit is packed with nutrients and color.
Cane sugar is partially refined, but needed in certain recipes.

I tried agave cactus syrup, but it seemed a bit refined, and brown rice syrup, same thing. So I narrowed it down to this list of five. These are the most unrefined, mineral rich, nutrient dense. And cane sugar is needed in certain recipes just because molasses, maple syrup, honey, and fruit, don't work. Blackstrap molasses, dark maple syrup, and raw honey, spell minerals, minerals, and nutrients, plus fruit, and the cane sugar. These NCD Five Healthy Sugars™ are all you need for sweetener. And some organic stevia occasionally.

So back to our fiber. Do we subtract or do we not subtract? With the NCD we crunch the numbers both ways so we can see the meal and the percent macros with the fiber included and with the fiber subtracted. Then the rest is intuition. If the meal has fiber and not enough sugar, you'll be back at the refrigerator shortly after you've eaten. A 35-30% carb meal will make you lose fat a bit faster, but you may feel low energy. A 50-60% carb meal may make you feel like you need to get on the treadmill and burn off some calories. We will crunch the recipes both ways, regular and subtracted, and then look at the whole meal for a best estimate that targets 40% carbs. There's just no way to know EXACTLY whether you can subtract the fiber calories or not. But this is good, because it's making you pay more attention to your body signs. Your Internals.

CHAPTER 2

NCD Omega 3 Protocol™

You will take one 454g 16oz bag of Bush Creek flax seeds and aliquot it, (divide it up), into ten 2oz SKS glass jars with the screw caps, 46g each. If you didn't buy the SKS glass jars mentioned in the *ABC Water and the Number Crunch Diet*, you can grind 23g directly from the bag each time you prepare a shake, or you can grind 46g from the bag, and use 23g and store the remaining 23g in some sort of airtight container that you have. The one-pound bag contains about 460g of flax seeds, so, 10x46g=460g. They give you a few extra grams. It is important to verify the weight of the food products you will be using. The six-pack of french-bread rolls says one roll is 71 grams, but they consistently make them 85-91g, so you are getting 46 more carb calories than you might think. I was tricked by this "one roll 71g" on the label, until I checked it.

The flaxseed bag is opaque, so no light gets in, and it has a ziplock so you can reseal it. Store them in the refrigerator. The website says the seeds will last indefinitely if stored sealed, protected from light, in the refrigerator, unground. If you have one Flaxseed Shake per day, then you will finish the bag in 20 days, $1/20^{th}$ of the bag per shake. If you have 20 flaxseed shakes a month, then after one year you will have eaten 12 pounds of flax seeds! This is some serious omega-3 therapy. And of the highest quality, and consumed the most beneficial way, FRESHLY GROUND.

Contrast this with the vast majority of the population who aren't eating flax seeds at all, or properly. This, and all of your other JPM strategies will have you looking HYA – HALF YOUR AGE!!

Ok, so we aliquoted our bag of flax seeds into 10 x 46g, and each aliquot of 46g will yield 2 servings of 23g for a total of 20 shakes.

Now, our Nutrition Facts label was for 20g, but for our shake we will be using 23g. This is 3g more. Don't get scared, just watch how I do this.

$23/20 = 1.15$

We are going to multiply all our Nutrition Facts numbers by 1.15.

23g
E=110x1.15=126.5=127 calories
F=70x1.15=80.5=81 calories
total Fat=72x1.15=82.8=83 calories
SF=9x1.15=10.4=10 calories
Omega-3 = 34.2x1.15=39 calories
Omega-6 = 11.7x1.15=13 calories
Omega-9 = 16.2x1.15=19 calories
TF=0
Chol=0
Na=0
K=170x1.15=196mg
CHO=20x1.15=23 calories
f=48x1.15=55 calories
s=0
Prot=16x1.15=18 calories
T= 83+23+18 = 124 calories

Are you okay? Some people are terrified of math. It's okay. It's just new at first, and then it's mindless repetition. Remember, you'll be miles ahead of the average person after a while when it comes to number crunching. Chances are, it will spill over into other areas, like, for example, you may stop forgetting where you put your car keys.

We will do this again, so no worries. But when you divide up a package of food, you have to recalculate the nutrition facts to match your new serving size. That's all we did.

Notice that the Nutrition Facts label gives you the fat in calories, F, but then it also gives you the fat in grams, Total Fat. This is another place where you will see a little discrepancy. In the above, the F = 81 but the total F = 83.

The new Nutrition Facts label will no longer have the F, (fat in calories), listed. So if you want to know the number of calories of fat, you will have to take the Total Fat in grams and multiply it by 9. Removing the Fat Cals is a bad move. If I pick up meat lasagna and the calories are 420 and the fat cals are 210, that tells me easily and quickly that the product is 50% fat, it goes back on the shelf.

When it comes to calculating the T, Total Calories at the bottom, I will use the total Fat in grams x9 number. So, 83+23+18=124 calories. The E at the top was 127. As you get comfortable with the label you will see how you can double-check their numbers and see discrepancies. Most of the time it's just slight.

Now let's go deeper with the numbers. Recall our example from the *ABC Water and the Number Crunch Diet*, Chapter 57, "Crunch Time!" If I have $1.00 total and I have 4 dimes, what percent of my money is dimes? 0.40/1.00=0.40x100=40%

If I have 83 fat calories, and 124 total calories, what's the percent fat? 83/124x100=67%

If I have 23 carb calories and 124 T calories, what's the percent carbs? 23/124x100=18.5% or 19% rounded off.

If I have 18 prot cals and 124 T cals, what's the percent protein? 18/124x100=15%

The marcos are 19 67 15. It should add up to 100 or 100%, but we rounded up twice, so 19+67+15=101. No biggie. If your three macro percents add up to 102, you made a calculation error, recrunch.

So flax seeds are 67% fat or about 2/3rds fat, as we would expect from seeds. They have some protein 15% and some carbs 19%.

Now most labels won't have a breakdown of omega 3 6 9, but this is an omega food, high in omega-3, so they have the three plant fats listed.

Our 23g serving of flaxseed has 39 calories of omega-3. What's the percent? 39/124x100=31%

FLAX SEEDS ARE 31% OMEGA 3 !!!!!!!!!!!!!!!!

Flax Seeds are almost 1/3rd Omega 3 !!!!!!!!!!!!!!!!!

Now are you getting it? Do you see how this is so critical to your diet? This is THEE way to get fresh stable U-shaped omega-3 fat.

DHA and EPA from cod liver oil, and Omega-3 from Flax Seeds.

Chia seeds are #2 and Hemp seeds are #3 for omega-3 content. I've never tried chia seeds, but they are imported from Mexico, South America, and Australia, and I would rather support my North and South Dakota organic flaxseed farmers. On page 53, Udo Erasmus, the PhD fat expert, states in *Fats That Heal Fats That Kill*, that hemp seeds contain only trace amounts of THC, tetrahydrocannabinol, cannabis, marijuana, but it is possible that it could show up in a urine drug screen. None-the-less, hemp seeds are loaded with minerals, good fat, and nearly 25% protein. You will enjoy an 8oz bag of raw organic hemp seeds with the NCD Orange Chicken™ recipe.

Your next sources of omega-3 are nuts, walnuts being the highest, but nowhere near the amount found in flax seeds. So, flax seeds win. And the NCD Flaxseed Shake™ is the ideal way to consume them.

The omega-6 percent in a 23g serving is 13/124x100=10%.
The omega-9 percent in a 23g serving is 19/124x100=15%.

Now what if we wanted to convert our 39 calories of omega-3 into grams? What would we do? Well, we used x9 to go from grams to calories, so it's divide by 9 to go back. 39/9=4.3g omega-3.

So each shake has 4.3g of omega-3 fat. This would be like 4.3 very large fish oil or salmon oil capsules, 1000mg each. Now, fish oil and flax are not the same, but this is just to give you an idea of how much 4.3 grams of omega-3 fat is. If you were taking 1000mg flax oil capsules, then one shake would have 4.3 capsules. Most people can't stomach all those capsules. Plus the oil is refined from the seeds, so you are losing nutrition, and gaining contaminants and rancidity.

The NCD says, eat as close to the original food as possible. In this case, eat the actual seeds, ground fresh.

I tried flaxseed oil, I didn't like it. And it spoiled quickly. That's the key trait of omega-3 fat, and fish oil. They're unstable fats.

So you have all the advice givers saying "eat more omega-3s" and never giving you exactly how to do it. Here it is.

JPM – from Advice to Results™

The advice givers also repeatedly say "Healthy Fats". If you've read *ABC Water and the Number Crunch Diet*, you know inside and out, the difference in fats and what a healthy and unhealthy fat is. It says right on the front of the book "new dietary fat categories". Read the book. It's a compilation of nearly 100 books that I've read in the past 13 years, each author having their own specialized area of health knowledge, and I've synergized that knowledge into a completely new area – Selfcare Protocols.

Lastly, our saturated fat is 10 calories per 23g serving shake. What is the percent? 10/124x100=8%

So, as you can see, the fat in flax seeds is 31% omega-3, 10% omega-6, 15% omega-9, and 10% saturated. God made this food for a specific purpose in MIND. Omega-3

Chapter Endnote
Coming up, you are going to see "less-than" and "greater-than". Initially, I spelled them as two separate words, but when I saw Wikipedia spelling them with hyphens, it occurred to me that, yes, we say it as a unit, and it sounds better as "lessthan" rather than "less than". Grammarians will disagree, oh well.

Also, you may have noticed that when there's a quotation within a sentence, that I place the comma on the outside of the quotation mark. Many writers and grammarians say you should place the comma inside the quotation. However, this gives the impression that the comma is part of the quotation. I keep my quotations "clean", and place the comma on the outside. Sorry grammarians.

Lastly, the word "thee" means you. Unfortunately, dictionaries don't have a word for "thē", the with a long e. When you say "the" with a long e, people understand this to mean "exclusively". Perhaps one day, dictionaries will update their definition of "thee" to say, 16th century "you", modern day "exclusively", or "only".

Page 264, *ABC Water and the Number Crunch Diet*
EPA = Eicosapentaenoic = i-co-sa-penta-en-no-ic Acid
DHA = Docosahexaenoic = doe-co-sa-hexa-en-no-ic Acid

Use those words in a sentence at your next employee potluck and you'll gain a whole new look of respect.

And then when they ask you why you don't refer to them as Omega-3s. Tell them, flax, chia, and hemp seeds have three double bonds whereas EPA and DHA have 5 and 6 double bonds. They're not the same molecules, and although they have overlapping roles, they also have uniquely different functions.

11

CHAPTER 3

Milk & Ellen White

I like to keep the chapters on the short side so that you stop and let it sink in. It's when you stop to ponder, that's when your mind starts planning how it can add this into your lifestyle.

Now recall that omega-3 can convert to DHA and EPA fish oil, our good hormones. The rate is small, 2.7%, but better than nothing. So our flaxseed shake with its 39 calories 4.3 grams of omega-3 can make about 116mg of EPA. This would be about $1/5^{th}$ of a teaspoon of cod liver oil. Not very much, but at least it's something. This is why we need both, flax and fish oil. Flax for membranes and fish oil for hormones. At one time they referred to flax seeds as "vegetarian fish oil", but it doesn't convert enough.

On the other hand, this is still uncharted territory, and there may be people who can convert flax omega-3 into fish oil DHA EPA at 10-20-30%. The great news is that omega-3 can convert to fish oil.

This again is why we do not call fish oil omega-3. Nor do we use the words "mono" and "polyunsaturated". Chapter 49 ABC NCD, dietary fats defined.

NCD Edible Fats™
3 6 9 plants
saturated animal fat and coconut oil
fish fat

Come on America! And the rest of the world! Get on board!
Imagine what could happen if people stopped consuming fryer oil?

2. Raw Milk
I buy mine at Lassen's Health Foods and from Organic Pastures
Dairy in Fresno, California. Thank you to both of these great
companies for fighting to keep raw milk on the shelves. In fact,
more people are buying it than ever before. This milk is so
beneficial. Read their website at www.organicpastures.com, it's
very very impressive. The founder/owner invented a mobile
milking machine so he can milk the cows out in the pasture and not
in a barn. I am sure you've seen pictures of some dairies. You
can't label all milk as bad. People that do that are just dumb. Raw
milk is good food – "Time Test" passed.

The label says, "We don't pasteurize or homogenize this perfect
raw food." It also boasts that it's a natural source of good bacteria
probiotics, so by drinking this milk I have no need for probiotic
supplementation. Good gut flora is essential to good health. Raw
milk provides this. It's USDA certified organic, meaning, no
hormones, no antibiotics in the feed, no sewer sludge used to grow
the feed, et cetera. That "sewer sludge" that Los Angeles ships up
here for nonorganic farming is about as good a reason as any to buy
organic. And if the spray pesticides and GMOs weren't bad
enough, now they want to irradiate the food to extend the shelf life.

I hope you can see the difference in the two types of food available
for you to eat. Normal traditional food made in line with nature
and God, and the other being man's way, adulterated, and seems to
be getting freakier with every passing few years. I bought some
eggnog a few years ago and the word "Cloned" was on the carton.
It read, "Not from cloned dairy." And it wasn't a joke. It was a
serious statement on the container. God help us if that's where
we're heading.

The raw milk from Organic Pastures does come in a plastic jug, but
this conscientious company has informed its customers that "Our
plastic bottles are free of BPA, bisphenol A, and no phthalates,

plasticizers." This is such a great company. All dairy producers should model themselves after this company. Berkeley Farms is another brand I buy sometimes, if I buy regular milk. It tastes good and I don't ever have a reaction. The company was established in 1910, so I like that it's been around for more than a century, and it says "Passionate about Purity" on the label. There's that "Purity" thing again. Even the milk producers are chiming in on it. Why? Because HEAVY METAL CONTAMINATION, or any and all sorts of contamination and pollutants and things that shouldn't be in your food and supplements are getting in. Pay attention to Purity. That's my advice. And know who you are buying from. And know the history of the companies you buy from.

"Oh, it's vegetable oil spread now, it's okay, it's not like the old margarine." Oh really.

And soft drink machines selling a 20oz cola for $1.00 that cost maybe 5 cents to make, what do you think of a company like this?

Vote with your dollars. Vote out the bad and vote in the good.

Raw milk also provides raw proteins, unheated, undenatured. The NCD is big on raw, aim for 80% raw and 20% cooked, and only cooked to MW (medium-well) or 3/4ths done, then allow it to finish cooking off heat to just right. We don't want rogue misshapened denatured proteins activating our immune system.

I can tolerate most brands of regular milk, (pasteurized homogenized), but there is one brand that consistently gives me bad GI reactions. This is dirty dairy milk. Cow butt bacteria is getting into the milk. Yuck. Bad Bacteria. I won't tell you the brand, but just be aware that there are many different kinds of cow's milk. Find a good one and start drinking it.

You will need a half gallon, 64oz, of whole milk for the recipe.
Nutrition Facts
1cup 240mL
servings per container 8

E=150cal
F=70cal
total Fat=8g x9=72cal   47%
SF=5g x9=45cal
TF=0
Chol=30mg
Na=105mg
CHO=12g x4=48cal   32%
f=0
s=12g x4=48cal
Prot=8g x4=32cal   21%
T=152

Okay, so 72+48+32=152 calories total. Our E at the top is 150, so it's close. F=70 and we calculated 72. Notice I placed the percent macros out to the right a bit, 47% fat 32% carbs 21% protein.

Try crunching them. 72/152x100=47% fat, 48/152x100=32% carbs, 32/152x100=21% protein.

0.5 rounds up, and 0.49 rounds down. Standard math rule.

Recall that our NCD Emergency Meal™ is 2% milk, 16oz is a snack, 250 calories, and one quart would be a meal, ~500 calories.

Whole milk is of course more milk fat. It's 32 47 21. Higher in milk fat and lower in protein and lower in carbs. This is a weight-gain food because the 32% carbs is all sugar. That sugar raises insulin and the whole thing gets converted into body fat.

Our 2% milk is more macro balanced. It was very close to the target 40 30 30, it was 38 33 29, see page 274 of the ABC NCD.

The higher protein, 29%, and lower fat, 33%, makes this less of a weight gainer. Although, you can still gain weight from 2% milk because all the carbs are sugar carbs. So you just drink it slower. Take it to your desk and drink it over an hour, a one-hour infusion. Then it becomes a nice long healthy satisfying meal. With an added benefit of minerals and hydration. A cow's sole purpose on this planet is to chew green grass all day long to make milk for humans. Chickens make eggs. How can you deny these foods?

I am going to speak to the Seventh-Day Adventists for a moment. Now I am a big believer in SDA principles and teachings. I even installed my own Glory Star satellite dish. For $200 you get FREE television for the rest of your life. Pay for the dish and pay nothing after that, no monthly charge, Great Deal! Glory Star satellite TV programming by the Three Angels Network, www.3ABN.org.

Toss your current TV provider in the trash, pay no monthly fees, and get better quality television. They will teach you about real history, real news, and, well, the real God. I'm not apologizing for that one.

So my Beef with SDA is this. Here's where they got it wrong about vegetarianism. Ellen White, the author and teacher of SDA principles, was ill. So she switched to an all fruit-and-vegetable diet and got well. Here's where today's SDAs get it wrong.

The all fruit-and-vegetable diet is for when you are ill.™

If you are not ill, you should be eating plants and animals.™

A healthy person can eat and tolerate all kinds of foods. It's also referred to as a "steel gut". A weak person can't eat this and can't eat that. That's not a healthy person.

Ellen White promoted veganism because she was ill and it made her well. Basically, she balanced her acid-base balance. She stocked up her alkaline reserves. She could have done the same thing by drinking the ABC Water for a source of bicarbonate base.

Seventh-Day Adventists misinterpret this to mean, that healthy people should eat a vegan diet. No. Sick people should eat a vegan diet. It's an alkaline diet, and most sickness symptoms are rooted in what? What? What is the root of most sickness and disease? Low alkalinity and high acidity in the body.

ALKALINE DEFICIENCY™
If you've read ABC NCD then you get this. Yay! You get it!

But not just "yay you get it", but "yay you get THE REASON WHY YOU DON'T FEEL WELL AND YOU'RE AGING."

ALKALINE DEFICIENCY ALKALINE DEFICIENCY ALKALINE DEFICIENCY

Never mind alkaline foods, just eat according to the NCD and track your urine pH to see where you're at – Chapter 10 ABC NCD.

So my fellow SDAs, you misinterpreted Ellen White's situation. The vegetarian diet is the "Get Well" diet. If you are well and healthy, then your next goal should be to become fit; strong flexible muscles with a great cardiovascular system, a gymnast, a diver, speed skater, hurdler. That's going to take some protein, 30%. Beans are 40% protein, but lean chicken, tuna, fish, turkey, and ham are 90-100% protein, lean pork chops are 75% protein, and lean beef is 2/3rds protein.

So there you have it. I just debunked the foundational dietary principle of the Seventh-Day Adventist religion. Ellen White used it because she was sick and it made her well. It's a Get-Well diet.

Ellen could have likely gotten better by supplementing with bicarbonate to fix her acidosis. But she likely needed the phytonutrients and the natural plant minerals and vitamins as well.

The two go hand in hand. God made both plants and animals. And we've been eating both for as long as time is recorded. Jesus ate fish with his bread, and I'll bet he drank cow's or goat's milk when he needed a quick snack.

We are going to use 1 cup 240mL 8oz of whole milk per flaxseed shake. So half a gallon will make eight shakes.

3. Fat Free Cottage Cheese

Sadly, the Trader Joe's brand now has "Natural Flavor". Shame Shame. So to get cottage cheese without Titanium Dioxide and Natural Flavor, you have to buy organic. Organic cottage cheese is now in the same price category as meat, fish, and poultry. And I have noticed that foods with protein cost more. It's like "someone" is making protein expensive for the average person. It's like "someone" is trying to get the average everyday person to eat inexpensive grains and junk foods. Does cottage cheese really need to be made with so much crap? Mono and diglycerides, locust bean gum, guar gum, xanthan gum, carrageenan, titanium dioxide, artificial flavor, natural flavor. And you will never convince me that "Natural Flavor" is raspberry flavoring extracted from fresh berries. Give me a break. The NCD says it's "Chemicals That Make You, and Me, Addicted To The Food Product." If it weren't for some of these "Exposers" we'd never know half the stuff that's going on in our world.

So plan on budgeting more for food in the future, as unadulterated food is going to be for the wealthy and the elite. Middle-class food for the middle class, and poor food for the poor. The New Normal.

Next Chapter Note

Throughout all JPM books, chemical compounds are hyphenated, just be aware that the standard rule is to spell them as separate words. If you say them together, with the hyphen, the sentence should flow better. Hopefully!

Also, there are two camps when it comes to hyphenating fractions. One group says, do not hyphenate if the denominator functions as a noun, only hyphenate if the fraction functions as an adjective. The other group says you should hyphenate all fractions regardless. I decided to go with the second camp, since, as a number, it's 2 slash 3, then as a written word it makes more sense to be two hyphen three. Also, as a noun, "two" is not modifying "thirds", the fraction is a unit, "two-thirds". While we're on the subject of math, if you see "~", read the word "about" or "approximately", ~10, about ten.

CHAPTER 4

NCD Mineral Shake™

Yes, this is likely to be the world's record for the longest recipe, more than 20 pages and 4 chapters. Hey, I did say that the NCD would have you looking at the foods you are eating with greater insight. That means detail.

For our 8-shake recipe we will need 4 lbs of nonfat cottage cheese, either 4x1 lb containers or 2x2 lb containers. (454g x4 or 907g x2)

The Nutrition Facts are for ½ a cup 113.5 grams.
I am going to multiply it by 2, so,
1cup 227g
E=160
F=0
total Fat=0   0%
SF=0
TF=0
Chol=0
Na=780mg cottage cheese contains a significant amount of salt
CHO=8g x4=32cal   22%
f=0
s=8g x4=32cal
Prot=28g x4=112cal 78%
T=144cal

So our NFCC is 78% protein. A good way to get protein. It's also a pretty high source of salt. Probably not the good kind, unrefined with natural minerals intact, but rather the white refined tablesalt, or the sodium-phosphate salt. The organic TJs brand has just as much salt. The NCD aims for Na to be <1g per meal. Keeping in mind that salt added is not the same as salt found naturally in the food. The one cup of raw milk has 105mg of naturally-occurring salt, not salt added during manufacturing.

If I have five meals a day, then my maximum salt intake would be 5 grams, naturally occurring and unnaturally added. If the meal has 1300mg of salt, Na=1300, then I do notice a slight thirst sensation after eating it. You would be hard-pressed to find a restaurant meal with less-than 1000mg or 1g of salt. This is why the waitress brings water to the table. You're going to need it later after you finish eating. Foods that contain salt naturally, don't make me thirsty. It's the added salts that make a person thirsty. Again, one word, salt, but lots of different varieties.

Some NCD meals have very little salt, so, by the end of the day, my intake for Na is less-than 3000mg 3g, which is the allowable recommended limit for a 2500-calorie a day diet. And then if you subtract the natural-occurring salt from that 3000mg then my daily "added salt" or "bad salt" is closer to 1500-2000mg, or less.

Chicken breast with the 15% solution is pumped full of sodium-phosphate salt. This and all the other "bad salts" are what raises blood pressure. MSG, monosodium glutamate, sodium phosphate, sodium pyrophosphate, sodium diacetate, you might as well just take a gun and blow your brains out because that is what these sodium salts are doing to the neurons in your head. Sorry, that was a bit strong. But my publisher suggested adding violence to sell more books. Read up on Excitotoxins and you'll see what I mean.

4. And our last ingredient, Molasses.
But as I have discovered, not just any molasses. It has to be Blackstrap and ideally Plantation brand. At the bottom of the Nutrition Facts label lists a few minerals, and what I discovered is, the well-known Grandma's brand that I purchased, because it was

cheaper, lacks minerals. The label says that a 1T serving has 2% of the RDA of calcium and 2% of the RDA of iron. You would think that molasses being unrefined sugar would contain more than that. Well, it does. But not this brand. I then bought the Plantation brand at the healthfood store and a 1T serving has 20% the RDA of calcium and 20% the RDA of iron. That's ten-times more calcium and iron than the regular grocery-store brand. This is why the healthfood store is so much better. It's the details. The devil is in the details, and the devil somehow removed 90% of the minerals. If calcium and iron are ten-times higher in the Plantation brand then you can assume all the other minerals are also ten-times higher. Conversely, if Grandma's brand has 90% less, 2% instead of 20% calcium and iron, then you can assume it has 90% less of all minerals. Maybe it's the soil, or perhaps it's the refining. The organic blackstrap molasses had 10% the RDA for calcium and 15% the RDA for iron and 8% the RDA for magnesium.

Whatever the reason for the difference in mineral content, I suggest you look for one with high minerals, 10-15-20% and not 2%, as the reason we are using this product is for sweetener and for the minerals.

I chose the nonorganic Plantation brand blackstrap unsulphured molasses, 15 fl oz, 442 mL, that came in a glass bottle for $8.49. This is four times as much money as the one in the one-gallon jug at Smart & Final, but without the minerals, you're just getting sugar. So now you know.

You will be pouring 360g of this molasses into your Ninja Blender, divided by 8 servings = 45g of molasses per shake.
E=90
F=0
total Fat=0   0%
SF=0
TF=0
Chol=0
Na=21
K=1286mg this is a high potassium mineral food, good

CHO=94cal   100%
f=0
s=94cal
Prot=0   0%
T=94cal
429mg Calcium
7.7mg Iron

The Nutrition Facts label is for 1T tablespoon 21g.
E=42
Na=10
K=600
CHO=11g
s=11g
Calcium 20% of RDA
Iron 20% of RDA

The RDA for calcium is 1000mg, so 20% is 200mg.   There is 200mg of calcium in 1T 21g of this blackstrap molasses. Nice.

The RDA for iron is 18mg, so 20% of 18 is 18x0.20=3.6. There is 3.6mg of iron in 1T 21g of this blackstrap molasses. Good.

Since our recipe uses 45g per serving, I divided 45/21=2.14, and multiplied all the numbers on the nutrition facts by 2.14.

So E=42x2.14=90cal, Na=10x2.14=21mg, K=600x2.14=1286 etc.

By using this brand of molasses, our shake has 429mg of calcium and 7.7mg of iron.   Almost half your RDA for both of these minerals. There's your nutrition. That your body needs.

Here's your clue.   If you see lots of potassium, then you can assume there are lots of the other minerals as well. My Grandma's brand molasses had 110mg of potassium per 1T, and my Plantation brand has 600mg of potassium per 1T.

Wouldn't it be great if we could have mineral data on the food label so we could see what kind of soil it was grown on and how much refining was done in the making of the food product?

Take some time to review the number crunching we just did. How if your label serving size says 1T 21g and you will be using 45g per Flaxseed Shake, how you have to do 45/21=2.14 and multiply all the numbers on your food label by 2.14, and in the case of the flax seeds we used 23g instead of 20g and did 23/20=1.15 and multiplied the entire label by 1.15. Get comfortable with that.

So our three molasses products are:
A. Grandma's brand – not blackstrap
B. Organic blackstrap
C. Plantation brand – blackstrap, not organic

Notice that I chose the nonorganic brand. For three reasons.
1. it had the highest calcium and iron percents
2. it came in glass
3. it had the lowest carbs

	Container	Calcium	Iron	Carbs
A.	plastic	2%	2%	16g
B.	plastic	10%	15%	14g
C.	glass	20%	20%	11g

Do you see the superior molasses brand?

The Plantation brand came in glass, it had the highest percent calcium and the highest percent iron, and the lowest carbs, 11g.

This is a good company. Vote for them.

The organic molasses came in plastic, it had higher carbs, therefore more refined, sweeter, less robust, and therefore along with more refined comes less minerals, 10% calcium and 15% iron.

The regular-supermarket everyday common brand was higher still in carbs, 16g, with a lot less calcium and iron, more refined.

This took me half a day to analyze, but it means a whole lot to your Divine Intelligence that needs these nutrients to make your body work properly.

If you've read the ABC NCD then you are reading labels. Good. Now the next step is to study and analyze them.   This is your master's degree in number crunchology.

The 1 cup of milk in the flaxseed shake has 300mg of calcium, and the 1 cup of NFCC has 200mg of calcium, for a total of 500mg. The 23g of flaxseed has 69mg of calcium, so that's 569mg. Now add to this the 429mg of calcium in the molasses, and you get 998mg of calcium.   This shake has ~1000mg of calcium, your recommended daily allowance (well it's RDV now, recommended daily value).

Now if this shake is packed with your RDA of calcium then it's likely to be packed with your RDA for magnesium, zinc, copper, chromium, and all of your other minerals as well. It could just as easily be called the NCD Mineral Shake™. This may be the longest recipe in history, but for a reason. It's packed with nutrition. And we've nearly forgotten about the reason for this shake in the first place, the omega three content! Plus it has 30% protein. This recipe is a masterpiece! Plus it tastes good.

All those people who put kale in their shakes, YUCK. Don't put greens in a shake, because no amount of sugar will make it taste good. They make these shakes on TV and the people take one sip of it and leave the rest. They don't even drink their own shakes! Eat your greens first thing when you get up and get them out of the way, and eat them alone, the NCD Leafy Greens Protocol™, page 250 ABC NCD.

Blending greens into a shake is just about the dumbest thing I've seen people do. You're just asking for Gross.

The NCD Shake Mistake!™

CHAPTER 5

NCD Secret Ingredient™

Time to make a batch of 8 shakes. Are you ready! Grab your Ninja! I hope you bought or already own one. I have the Pro System 1100. It has 6 blades, 2 at the bottom, 2 in the middle, and 2 at the top. You will need all these blades plus the 1100 watts of power to convert the cottage cheese into liquid protein.

NCD Secret Ingredient™
LIQUEFIED Nonfat Cottage Cheese™

This is worth the price of this book, in my opinion.

Have you noticed there's no protein powder in this shake, or any of my recipes? I don't own protein powder. Now I am not against it, but SOOOOO many diet books use protein powder to raise the protein content of their shakes. I came up with a natural way.

Take nonfat cottage cheese and blend it in your Ninja, and voila! You have liquid casein and whey protein – From Food.™

I've never seen or read or heard of anyone doing this, JPM – *Your First Choice for Selfcare Strategies.*

Nonfat cottage cheese is 78% protein. The rest is 22% lactose milk sugar. This 78% protein content is better than a lot of protein powders on the market, some of which are only 40-50% protein or less.   A friend of mine had one and it was so sweet.   When I crunched the numbers, it was 81% carbs sugar, 12% protein, and 7% fat.   Can you say "Protein Powder Scam"?   You get more protein in a peanut-butter sandwich.

You have to crunch the numbers to see what you are really eating, and paying for.™

So none of the NCD recipes, NONE, have protein powder in them. And yet they all contain 30% protein. I know, it's amazing.

Although I am not against using protein powder, (like the one I referred to on page 93 of the main book), it is a refined product from milk, and it is dry, dehydrated, and a bit lifeless. If I do start to use it, it will only be a small 25-calorie serving added to about 4oz of raw milk, taken before bed to supply my body with amino acids for muscle synthesis while I sleep. Not as the protein portion of a meal or shake.

So, place the blade into your Ninja pitcher and then add your two quarts of NFCC. Place it on the scale and press "on", it will read zero. Add 360g of your crude blackstrap molasses. Secure the lid and blend on #2 for 5 minutes. Set a timer. The Ninja has three settings, low, medium, and high. Since we are blending for 5 minutes, I use the medium speed to protect the motor. It's smooth looking within 2-3 minutes, but I like my liquid cottage cheese to be super smooth, completely blended.

While the timer is ticking, get 8 of your 32oz SKS glass jars with the screw caps. See page 24 of the main book for where to purchase them.

Now, you will want to record the weight of your empty Ninja pitcher with blade and lid. Mine's 1137 grams. So when my five minutes are up, I stop the blender, remove the pitcher from the base and place it on the scale. Using your calculator, subtract 1137g from the weight, and this is the weight of the pitcher's contents. For me it's about 3329g – 1137g = 2192g divided by 8 = 274g. So each of my servings is going to be 274g. See how I did that? The blender contains the whole batch of 8 servings, and the contents weighs 2192g, so 2192g/8=274g. So now remove the blender lid, place one of your 32oz jars on the scale, press "tare" to zero it, and pour 274 grams into the jar. Repeat 6 more times. So you now have 7 jars filled and the remaining amount in the blender pitcher is your 8th serving. Pour out as much as you can into the 8th jar. Now place the pitcher on the scale and add 240g of the whole milk. Place the pitcher lid on tight and shake it up-and-down to dissolve the NFCC from the walls of the pitcher. Pour it into your 8th jar. Cap it. Add 240g of the whole milk to each of the remaining 7 jars and cap them. Refrigerate them all. You now have 8 jars of molasses shake. Clean up.

Each of these 8 jars has 1 cup of whole raw milk, 1 cup of NFCC, and 45g of blackstrap molasses.

Time to make a Flaxseed Shake.

Take your 2oz SKS jar with the 46g of flax seeds that we aliquoted earlier. Add the entire 46g to your coffee grinder and grind it for 10-15 seconds, shaking the coffee grinder up-and-down a bit to prevent the flax from sticking to the sides. If you grind longer than 15 seconds your flax seeds will begin to stick to the insides, creating a slight paste. So 10-15 seconds of grinding only. This also mixes the seed so that there are no unground seeds when you are done. Just grinding on the table doesn't mix the seeds enough. So just hold the grinder in your hands and gently shake it as you grind and count to 10. That's it. Stop. Your 46g of flax seeds should be perfectly ground with no sticking to the interior. It will turn into seed butter if you keep grinding it.

While holding the grinder and cap, turn the grinder upside down, tap the side of the grinder with the heel of your hand to dislodge the flax, then slide the grinder out from the cap. You now have 46 grams of ground flaxseed in your cap, cup. Ingenious, I know.

Place the 2oz SKS jar on the scale, zero it, then spoon in 23g of the ground flaxseed. Cap and refrigerate it. This is your second aliquot/serving for later.

The remaining ground flax in your cap cup, is your 23g serving for your shake right now. Add it to the jar of NFCC-milk-molasses. Cap & Shake. Shake it hard with both hands for about 20 seconds. This is your ab workout for the day. Seriously. If you hold your core tight, and shake that jar for 30-45 seconds, you will be out of breath and have sore, tight, rock-hard abs the next day. Do it!

There's a dumbbell called the "Shake Weight". I have two of them. Don't laugh. They work. You won't get huge muscles, but you will definitely wake them up and make them tight. So hold your core tight and shake that jar of your flaxseed shake as hard and as fast as you can for as long as you can. Then open the lid and reward yourself with a drink. Mmm!

Alternatively, you can replace the lid with the "lid with hole" and use your glass drinking straw, page 26 ABC NCD. When you are finished, add a little water to the jar and gently swirl it to wash off the insides so you don't waste any of this nutrition-packed meal.

It's 500 calories and 40% carbs 30% fat 30% protein.

You know, a word of caution about those protein-powder shake formulas. I know a guy who won second place in a weight-loss contest and received a $5000 home gym. A year later he blew up like a balloon, gaining it all back and then some. He said he stopped drinking the protein-powder shakes because it was costing him $100+ a month. Do you see the connection? Cheating never gets you anywhere but back where you started, or worse. Sadly, these companies never tell you what happens when you stop drinking their weight-loss shakes. So now he's in worse shape than before with no knowledge or understanding to get him going in the right direction. It was short lived glory. And a waste of a year.

Four Ingredients

1. NFCC – for lean protein
2. Unrefined sugar – for minerals and sweetness
3. Raw Milk – for protein, fat, carbs, minerals, and PROBIOTICS!
4. Flax Seeds – for omega-3 fat and other fats and fiber

For anyone who's looking to make a little pocket money, you can open a ClickBank account for free, just click on the affiliate link near the bottom of my homepage, and add a link to your emails or tweets. Have the person go through your link to the homepage and when they purchase any book, you'll be paid. Ka-Ching! You won't get rich, but if you want to help people, refer them to the website and get paid something. Who knows what could happen if/when alkalinity goes mainstream!

So with regard to protein powders, word to the wise, don't assume they are harmless or chemically free. You really have no way of knowing for sure.

To obtain the final numbers for our Flaxseed Shake we simply add each line together from each of our four food items.

E=127+150+160+90=527 calories

F=81+70+0+0=151 calories　　　　　　　　　29.4%

total Fat=83+72+0+0=155 calories　　　　　　30.2%

SF=10+45+0+0=55 cal

Omega-3 = 39 cal

Omega-6 = 13 cal

Omega-9 = 19 cal

TF=0+0+0+0=0

Chol=0+30+0+0=30mg

Na=0+105+780+21=906mg

K=196+NA+NA+1286=1482mg

CHO=23+48+32+94=197 cal　　　　　　　　38.3%

f=55+0+0+0=55 cal

s=0+48+32+94=174cal=33.9%

Prot=18+32+112+0=162 cal　　　　　　　　31.5%

T=124+152+144+94=514 cal

LOTS of numbers! I know. Two years from now you will have a

complete handle on this. But for right now it scares you. At the beginning you just buy the food items, make the recipe, and divide it up (aliquot it). The numbers are already crunched. From here on, it's just repetition. You will see the same breakdown, just different numbers for different foods. It's ok ☺ .

Chapter Endnote
At the bottom of page 26 my pitcher's contents is 2192g, however, if you add the grams of each item, 907g for 2lbs cottage cheese x2 =1814g, plus 360g molasses = 2174g. This is 18g more, 2192-2174g=18g, because each container of cottage cheese is really 916g, they give you a few extra grams.

Also note that, 1lb=454g and 2lbs=907g, not 908g. This is because 1lb is really 453.6g, which rounds up to 454, but 453.6x2=907g.

You're becoming an expert already!

CHAPTER 6

KEY PROTEIN

Now let's examine some of the numbers for a closer look at the beauty of this shake meal.

Meal? Yes, a meal. On the far right of the previous page are the macronutrient percents, percent macros. What are they?

Fat = 30.2%
Carbs = 38.3%
Protein = 31.5%

38.3 30.2 31.5, or in whole numbers, 38 30 32.

Recall from the NCD book how we calculate it:
fat cals over Total cals = 155/514 x100 = 30.2%
carb cals over Total cals = 197/514 x100 = 38.3%
protein cals over Total cals = 162/514 x100 = 31.5%

Note also, that there are two percent fats. One using "Calories from Fat" on the nutrition facts label, noted as "F", and the other using "Total Fat in grams" from the nutrition facts label. They are about the same, 151 and 155, and when you crunch them you get 29.4% and 30.2%, about the same.

The carb percent of this meal shake is 38.3%. A bit lower than our target of 40% but that's because there's sugar in this meal and it's also a liquid meal. So, for a shake, a liquid meal, you don't want to go over 40% carbs, and better to keep it a bit under.

While we're at the carbs, let's look at the sugar. The NCD recipes aim at keeping the sugar calories to <100, less-than 100. This would mean that the percent sugar of the meal is <20%. See how I did that? Meals are 500 calories, 100 over 500 = 0.2 x100 = 20%.

This shake is 174 calories of sugar. Many of you are thinking, WOW, that's a lot of sugar. It is but it isn't. Look closer. 174 calories of sugar over 514 total calories x100 = 33.9%. This meal is about $1/3^{rd}$ sugar. Contrast this with a 12oz can of soda or juice that's 150 calories of 100% straight pure sugar, no fat, no fiber, no protein. This is where the learning comes in. The total sugar is important, but the percent sugar of the entire thing you are eating is equally if not more important – "Glycemic Load" page 188.

A 500-calorie meal with 200 calories of carbs, 40% carbs, and 100 calories of sugar, 20%, is just the right formula to keep your brain from falling asleep and your body from becoming lethargic. If those sugar and carb calories aren't there, you are going to be back in the kitchen or at the vending machine 60 minutes after eating.

Sugar Has A Function – Use It But Don't Abuse It™

Now for our liquid shake, this makes a great way to get proteins fats and carbs into your bloodstream after you just used them all up during your high-intensity workout. I drink half the shake immediately, and then take 20 minutes to drink the rest. If I haven't worked out, then I will drink it gradually over 30-45 minutes while doing errands or at my desk. From experience, I can tell you that I have never had a physiological insulin spike from this shake, not even if I drink the entire shake in 10 minutes. The 34%, one-third sugar, means that the other two-thirds is fat, protein, complex carbs, and fiber, all of which slow down the glycemic load of this shake meal.

There are two other shakes that I see people making that the NCD does not recommend.

#1. The high-fruit high-carb soy/almond/rice milk shake.

Well, we already know that soy milk and almond milk and all the other "milks" are not used in the NCD. We use raw milk, or a good-quality paho milk, pasteurized homogenized milk. Soy is high in plant estrogens and almonds are eaten as raw almonds, unrefined and very close to their original form, just missing their shells. And rice milk, well, where's the protein in rice? Unless they artificially fortify rice milk with protein. The NCD avoids artificial ingredients and manufacturing whenever possible.

This fruit and soy/rice/almond milk shake may contain a little plain yogurt, but most of the time not. Thus, making this shake high glycemic. I would estimate 2/3rds sugar or 75-80% sugar. This would cause an insulin spike, depending on the amount (total calories) consumed, and the speed of consumption.

Bottom line – It's not a meal. It's missing the 30% protein.

In fact, sometimes they add peanut butter to this high-carb shake. What does it turn into when you add peanut butter? DESSERT! It becomes a carbfat. This is why if you are following any other NON-Number Crunching Plan, you may be in big trouble.

You've got to crunch the numbers to see what you are really eating.

You think you are eating "Healthy" but you are simply eating dessert.™

35% fat with 55% carbs-sugar and 10% protein is dessert, even if it's organic nut butter and fresh banana and blueberries. Sorry.

#2. The protein-powder shake.

Here, the recipe calls for protein, because the maker of the recipe understands that you need protein to be there or else it's a dessert.

This person is at least a step more informed than the person above.

Unfortunately, protein powders are not the way to go. They are manufactured. And even though Nutrabio.com makes an excellent protein powder (see ABC NCD), it shouldn't be consumed daily as part of a meal. I've heard of bodybuilders who are allergic to protein powders because their bodies are so overloaded with the stuff. This is why it's important to rotate your foods. By building a Recipe Repertoire. You've heard of P90X and Muscle Confusion, well, think of dietary confusion.

Dietary Confusion™ – where you continually change what you eat.

Most bodybuilders eat the same ten foods week-in week-out, brown rice, broccoli, chicken breast, tuna, sweet potatoes, eggs, egg whites, steak, berries, and protein powder. Then come Saturday night they eat pizza and beer. Well, as long as you're happy and it works for you. For the rest of us, we have the Number Crunch Diet™. And we have the NCD Hawaiian Pizza! Check it out on YouTube! Subscribe!

No one has ever figured out a way of getting casein and whey protein from food, until now.

LIQUEFIED NONFAT COTTAGE CHEESE™

78% PROTEIN – You heard it here first.

Nonfat Greek yogurt is 76% protein, which is good, but it has a mild sour taste, whereas nonfat cottage cheese is fairly neutral. I use greek yogurt in the NCD Pumpkin Cheesecake™ with a crushed almonds, walnuts, and dates pie crust. Another reason I don't use greek yogurt is because most brands have "live active cultures" so you have to be careful about how much you eat. One cup every day would likely be too much. Plus it's more expensive.

Anyway, the reason greek yogurt has become so popular is because of it's high-protein, but lucky for you, you've found a better way!

CHAPTER 7

The Numbers!

The NCD Flaxseed Shake™ is simple, four ingredients. But its amazing benefits are…are…well, there's just so many that it takes 46 pages to write! I am proud to say that this is the longest recipe in the history of the world – Because It's The Most Beneficial.

Moving on with our percent macros, we have 30.2% fat, 38.3% carbs, and the last one, 31.5% protein. This is why it's a meal. A Number Crunch Diet meal. Without that 30% protein, you are moving towards dessert. Higher protein and less carbs and more fat, means you are heading towards the low-carb ProFat Atkins diet. And as explained in the *ABC Water and the Number Crunch Diet*, this strategy only works for a while, as one day your carb cravings and urges are going to overtake you and boom!, you begin a backward trek to where you originally started.

I encourage you to purchase a copy of *ABC Water and the Number Crunch Diet* as it will explain in full detail why the low-carb and high-carb diets are not going to get you to where you want to be in the long term. They might, but for many they don't, and then you just feel more hopeless about getting control of your body weight, and the clock ticks on.

Take control of the numbers and you Take control of your weight.

This is key for bodybuilders and athletes who are looking to gain weight and muscle. Your coach will tell you to eat more calories, but be careful, those calories may not turn into muscle, and then you have a heck of a time getting the weight off if you don't understand the numbers.

Fiber. This shake has 55 calories of fiber, fantastic! That's 55/514 x100 = 10.7 or 11% fiber. This shake is more than 10% fiber. In fact, it's almost half the RDV recommended daily value of 30g. Okay, did you calculate it? I gave you two different units of measure in that last sentence, 55 calories and 30 grams. Fiber is a carbohydrate, so the conversion is x4. Going the other way, from calories to grams, it's /4, divide by 4. So, 55/4=13.75g. Half of your RDV of 30g of fiber per day is 15, so this shake has nearly half your recommended daily fiber intake.

All of you that read ABC NCD surely got that. For the rest of you, BUY THE BOOK!! It will help you more than all the other stuff you spend money on.

Sodium. The NCD likes to keep the sodium, Na, to <1g, or <1000mg. Recall that the < sign looks like an L for less-than. Then the other one, > is greater-than. I call these tidbits. I throw them in in hopes that you will learn other things besides diet. The ABC NCD has, in my opinion, many of these tidbit extras thrown in. Bits of wisdom too. Though I'm not claiming to be the real Messiah! Just the Selfcare Messiah, with tried-&-tested Strategies.

So sodium <1000mg, otherwise I find I get thirsty. Which just means you drink a glass of water 30 minutes after the meal if the sodium is 1300mg. If your meal Na is 1700 or 2000mg, expect your baseline blood pressure to go up ten points on the systolic, (top number), by the next morning. Repeated meals of 1500-1700-2000mg will snowball your systolic, until, uh-oh, you have a headache, and surprise, BP 180 over 95. Typically, the NCD recipes do not have this much sodium. When they do, like for example the NCD Beef Dip™, the recipe makes six meals, and you have one per day, and then you don't make that recipe again for six months. Plus, you balance out this high-sodium meal with low-sodium meals, and there are several very low-sodium meal recipes, and many others are <500mg. Cafeteria food and fastfood are loaded with sodium, and not the good kind. So make your own meals and watch your blood pressure go down.

Cottage cheese is a high sodium food, and this is where all the sodium is coming from in this recipe, sadly, sodium phosphate. The Trader Joe's organic cottage cheese has just as much sodium. But, we are under 1000mg, Na=906, and the sodium is not glutamate, MSG, so we're okay.

Potassium (K). This is not normally included in the nutrition facts, so the NCD doesn't usually include it either, however, what's great is that the K in this recipe is high, 1482mg. Why? Because the sugar ingredient is unrefined. Unrefined means that the minerals are still there. So you get to eat them, making them available for your Divine Intelligence to use within your body as it sees fit. The molasses contributes 1286mg of potassium. This is key. Because if you see that the mineral potassium is there and high, then you can assume it's unrefined and that many of the other minerals are there as well.

Refining takes out the minerals. Unrefining leaves them in.™

High potassium on a food label indicates the food is unrefined.™

An editor once corrected my writing, stating that I was using certain words incorrectly. I knew that. Unrefining is not a word. Microsoft underlines it in red, how could I not know? I use these "incorrect" versions of words to get them to stick, to get under your skin, to gnaw at the back of your head, so that the next time you are grocery shopping, you will pick up plain sugar or grade-A maple syrup, and something will spark, Unrefining Unrefining, and you will ask yourself, "Is what I am buying the most unrefined available?"

I just gave away my secret for getting something to stick and become a part of your life. (Hope it will continue to work.)

Aliquoting is also not a word. It's Unique to the Number Crunch Diet. Every company with an original product does this. You create unique words and features that are linked to your product. Bring a birthday cake to your job and six people will have six different serving sizes. An aliquot is a measured serving, a calculated serving, it's a Number-Crunched Serving.™

Aliquot – a number-crunched serving.™
Aliquoted – divided the whole into number-crunched servings.™

Aliquoting, the new term in dieting.™

So our potassium of 1482 nicely balances out our sodium of 906, and with a high potassium, we can feel comfortable knowing that the other nutrients and minerals are present as well, unrefining.

Cholesterol 30mg, nothing significant. But the NCD doesn't worry about dietary cholesterol. What! Why? Because the liver synthesizes (makes) cholesterol from excess carbohydrates and sugars. Dietary cholesterol in the body accounts for only 40% of your body's total cholesterol. 60%, more than half, of your body's cholesterol is being created by the liver from too much sugar. The NCD says that high cholesterol foods, like eggs, are good for you.

As amino acids are the building blocks of all your proteins and enzymes, cholesterol is the building block for all your steroid hormones. So rather than take steroids, eat eggs.

Saturated Fat. The NCD doesn't worry too much about this. We need it. But not a complete diet of saturated fat. All I am saying is, the media makes saturated fat out to be bad, because the average person is consuming 50% of their fats as saturated fats. But if you follow the NCD Dietary Fats Explained™, your saturated fat intake will be <30%. No need to dwell on saturated fat. This shake has 55 calories of SF. How many grams is that? Fat grams to calories is x9. Going the other way, then divide by 9, so 55/9=6 grams of saturated fat per shake. No cause for alarm. Pork ribs and nonlean beef and dairy have SF, so that's where you need to pay attention.

T Total calories at the bottom is 514, and E calories at the top is 527, so a bit of a discrepancy but a pass as far as matching goes. Note that there is no "T" on a nutrition facts label. We have added it to the bottom and calculated it by adding together our three foods, fat carbs protein. In this recipe it's 155+197+162=514. Always do this calculation to verify that your E calories at the top is correct. And you should do this with individual foods as well. You ABC-NCD readers will recall our dry powdered milk example, E=80 and T=80.

So what else? We covered %fat, %carbs, %protein, sugar, fiber, sodium, potassium, saturated fat, TF trans fat is zero, as always, per NCD rules, cholesterol, and total calories. Oh, Omega-3!

Just kidding. I didn't forget. I throw humor in here-and-there to keep you engaged. And to give your mind a break.

Here's where it gets exciting! And yes, I really do mean Exciting! You'll see why at the end.

Each shake has 39 calories of omega-3, 13 calories of omega-6, that's fine, we need some omega-6 as it is essential, we just don't want it from refined corn, soy, sun, and safflower oils, we want it from foods, corn on the cob, frozen organic corn, sunflower seeds, nuts, etc. We don't need to "seek out" omega-6. See ABC NCD. And lastly, 19 calories of omega-9 per shake, also known as OAP, Olives Avocado Peanuts. Omega-9 is a good fat and is included in the NCD, but it's not a "Seek Out" fat. Our two seek-out fats are, Omega-3 Flax and Cod Liver Oil fish fat.

So, 39 of 3, 13 of 6, and 19 of 9. 39 calories of omega-3 is the highest, by far. There is three times as much omega-3 as omega-6, 13x3=39, and twice as much omega-3 as omega-9, 19x2=38. So, do you see why you should be eating flax seeds? It's THEE source in the diet of all the foods available with the most amount of omega-3. And the NCD Flaxseed Shake Recipe™ is your way of consuming them. Jumper Publications & Media – from Advice to Results.

I make these plugs for my publications because I was up to my ears with advice from books and magazines and on television, with no real answers for exactly how to do that advice. So I came up with my own methods, or protocols. I hope you can appreciate how unique, simple, and loaded with nutrition this recipe is. And 30% protein with no protein powder! People will say, "That's impossible!" "You have to use protein powder to get that amount of protein, or egg whites." Trust me, and everyone else that's tried it, don't eat raw egg whites. Never mind, go ahead and try it!

So our 39 calories of omega-3 makes up 25% of the fat of this shake. The numbers are, 39/155 x100 = 25%, where 155 is the total number of fat calories. The entire shake is 7.6% omega-3 fat, 39/514 x100 = 7.6%. Our 39 calories of omega-3 is 4.3 grams of omega-3, 39/9=4.3g. (Fat grams to calories = x9. Going the other direction, fat calories to grams = /9.)

If you buy omega-3 eggs, chickens that have flaxseed added to the feed, you'll be paying about $3 for a dozen nonorganic eggs. This is double the price of regular eggs, and all they do is add flaxseed to the chicken's diet. These eggs have 225mg of omega-3 per egg. Your shake has the equivalent of 19 of these eggs, 4300/225=19. If you've read ABC NCD, then you know that 4.3g is 4300mg.

Your flaxseed shake is 1/20th of a pound of flax seeds. So if you had one shake per day, for three weeks, then skipped a week, by the end of the year you will have consumed TWELVE pounds of flax seeds. That would be equal to 1 Kg of omega-3 fat!!!!!!!!!!

Yes, 1 kilogram or 2.2 lbs, or 1,000,000mg, or 4444 omega-3 eggs.

39 calories omega-3 per shake times 20 shakes per pound times 12 bags (pounds) a year = 39x20x12=9360 calories of omega-3 per year, divided by 9 = 1040 grams per year, divided by 1000 = 1.04 kilograms Kg of omega-3 fat per year. There are 454g in one pound, so 1040g/454g=2.3lbs. That's 2.3 pounds of omega-3 fat per year. Your body will be quite happy with that. No deficiency. No dry skin. No countless other biological problems.

CHAPTER 8

NCD FSR Variations™

Now before I move on to the two variations of this shake, I regret to inform you that Bush Creek Organic Farms, the maker of this beautiful flaxseed, is no longer in business. I think they are selling their flax seeds to Arrowhead Mills. In the ABC Water book we talked about "voting with your dollars". You see, if you don't vote for these good farmers, they will disappear. And then one day, all we have for food are cereals, margarine, soft drinks, and ice cream. I'm serious. You need to seek out good companies and support them. The healthfood store, organic food, raw milk, organic flaxseed, independent researchers! If you don't give them some of your food-budget money, they won't be around in the future.

So I purchased 17 bags of Arrowhead Mills Organic Golden Flax Seeds, 14oz for $2.99. Great price, and the shipping is free if you spend $49, so 17x$2.99=$50.83. Bob's Red Mill sells the same thing in the 16oz size, but they also sell them ground. Don't buy them already ground, because why? The "U" shape of the fatty acids of omega-3 and fish oil DHA and EPA are very unstable. You grind them and eat them immediately. I will store my ground flaxseed 1-2 days in a sealed airtight container in the refrigerator, but not 4-5 days. Fish, eat it the same day you catch it.

The website is www.vitacost.com. I like this company already.

Whichever brand you buy, the amount is still 23g per shake.

NCD Maple Shake™

For the maple shake you are just going to substitute 275g of grade-B maple syrup for the molasses. Grade B is less refined than grade A, or light amber, and it will therefore have more minerals. I purchase mine at Trader Joe's and it's TJs brand, 32 fl oz, 1 quart, 946mL, for $16.99. But the price of maple syrup keeps going up, so what does that tell you? It's a valuable product.

Now, you will notice that the front label doesn't say how many grams. It lists the product by volume, 32floz, 1qt, 946mL milliLiters. So I have figured out the grams for you.

60mL = 78g

Should you ever encounter a product that doesn't list their food by weight, you will have to do some measuring to figure it out. But the NCD recipes have it all done for you.

So my TJs 100% Pure Maple Syrup Grade-B label reads:
1/4cup 60mL
servings per container = 16 (32oz ÷ 2oz ¼cup = 16)
E=200cal
F=0
total Fat=0g   0%
SF=0g
TF=0g
Chol=0mg
Na=5mg
CHO=53g x4 = 212 calories   100%
f=0
s=53g x4 = 212 cals
Prot=0g   0%
T=212

This product is also from Canada. Try to pick places where things are grown in the-middle-of-nowhere, Hawaii, Alaskan Salmon, North Dakota flax seeds. While driving up the I-5 freeway through

Central California, I noticed something I've never seen before. Several of the orchards had plastic tents over the crops. Dust, dirt and pollution falling on the crops is making them sick. Sadly whenever it rains, the first rain is full of dirt, almost like mud. Your car gets covered in dirt. Then the second day of rain it's cleaner, and the third day of rain is clean rain. So, look at the big picture when selecting foods. If air pollution is bad for people, it's bad for plants too. Coastal areas tend to be cleaner, and rural areas.

So our 275g of maple syrup gets added to our Ninja in place of the 360g of Plantation-brand blackstrap molasses. This means our batch of eight shakes will be 85g less (360-275=85). Dividing by eight, 85/8=10.6, so each shake will be about 10-11 grams less in weight when you go to aliquot it. So, for the molasses shakes you poured 274g into each of the eight 32oz glass jars, for the maple shake you'll pour 263g.

If you weighed your Ninja pitcher empty, then you can always weigh the Ninja pitcher with the NFCC-maple-syrup, and subtract the weight of the empty pitcher to get the weight of your shake batch. Then divide by 8 to get the grams per serving that you will pour. I posted on my refrigerator the weight of my empty Ninja pitcher with lid and it's 1137g. So I just weigh the entire pitcher with contents, subtract 1137, divide by 8 (servings), and that's my number, the number of grams I pour into each jar.

Each shake will have 34g of maple syrup.
E=88
Na=2
CHO=93
s=93

The CHO for the molasses is 94. So the maple syrup will result in essentially the exact same macro percents, 38 30 32, rounded off.

There's no point in crunching it all again. Just substitute 275g of maple syrup for the molasses and aliquot it into 8 servings of 263g. Oh, and Party On Down! Because this tastes delicious! No Kale!

The TJs maple syrup comes in plastic, and if you are a NCD reader then you are a professed and committed Plastiphobe. So I transfer my maple syrup to a one-quart one-liter glass amber bottle using a funnel, and then refrigerate it so that it lasts a long time without degrading, and since I use clean sterile technique when transferring it, I am assured of no bacterial or mold growth.

The 275g of maple syrup is equal to about 212mL. The container is 946mL, so 946/212=4.46 or 4.5. You can make 4.5 batches of this shake per 32oz container of maple syrup. I typically have this maple shake about once a month. So by the end of the year I've consumed about 2½ quarts of maple syrup. You will have no cravings for pancakes with syrup if you follow this protocol.

Your body doesn't want the pancakes, as it's just refined flour. What it wants are the minerals in the maple syrup. Unfortunately, if you eat pancakes at a restaurant you get ZERO minerals as maple syrup is way too expensive so they use pancake syrup, which is just HFCS and maple flavoring. Just like the little peel-off packets of strawberry jam is just sugar and red food dye. Read the label the next time, there's no strawberries in the ingredients, but they're allowed to call it strawberry. Go figure.

Word of warning. In the beginning when you drink this maple shake, your body will recognize the nutrition and say "More More Faster Faster". You are likely deficient in tree sap nutrients. Drink it slowly over 30-45 minutes so that you slow down the glycemic load. As time progresses and you've had say 2+ quarts in 12 months, then you won't feel that urge to drink it so fast.

Do you remember the following from page 159 of the ABC NCD?

What if much of the food you eat over and over again, and overeat, what if, your body's searching for something it needs? Well, not "what if", THAT'S EXACTLY WHAT'S HAPPENING.

Your eyes will see with new insight and you'll be a changed person after you read the book. A better person. A more informed person.

NCD Honey Shake™

Like molasses and maple syrup, honey is so good for you. It's a God food. Made by bees, not man. But there are better brands and kinds than others. I buy Trader Joe's Creamed Honey, 1lb, $4.49. It's 100% North American Clover Honey, Product of USA. The reason I buy it though is because it's UNfiltered and UNcooked. That's what is says on the label, "Unfiltered and Uncooked".

It's Raw Honey. And it's Unrefined.

Our nutrients are present and have not been removed or destroyed.

The honey is hard at room temperature. Hard as a rock. Liquid honey has been heated, "cooked". This liquid honey is now liquid for the life of the product. It's permanently changed. Someone I once worked with had never seen rock-hard honey before.

The other honey I sometimes buy is from Smart & Final, and it's Faraon-brand Honey With Comb. It's liquid honey but it has a big stick of the comb in it. The comb is delicious, not sweet, just chewy and fun to eat. I don't eat the comb alone as it's covered in the liquid honey, but I add it to the shake, (Ninja pitcher), and some of the pieces don't blend so there are a few bits of chewy honeycomb pieces in the shake.

The amount is the same for either honey you use. Add 232g of honey to your Ninja pitcher instead of the molasses. The raw hard honey may not blend smoothly, that is, some of the honey may fall to the bottom and not be blended into the shake. I am still trying to figure out how to prevent this from happening. So, what I do is, add the 232g to a glass bowl and microwave it for 30 seconds, then add it to the Ninja pitcher. I don't like doing this as it "cooks" my raw honey, but it's very minimal, and 30 seconds is just enough to soften it to a thick liquid. The honey will also soften to a liquid if you leave it in a warm area, (near a window on a sunny day). But until I get the hard chunks of honey to blend thoroughly, I am using the 30-second microwaving to soften it some. It doesn't get hot, it just softens it to a thick pourable liquid.

My TJs honey reads:
1T 21g
servings ~22 (it's a 454g container, so 454g/21g=21.6 servings)
E=60
F=0
total Fat=0   0%
SF=0
TF=0
Chol=NL (not listed, but cholesterol is only found in animal foods)
Na=0
CHO=17g=68cal   100%
f=0
s=16g=64cal
Prot=0   0%

Again, it's a 100% sugar food, like molasses, like maple syrup.

Each shake will have 29g of honey, 232g/8servings=29g.
E=83
CHO=94
s=88

Our CHO is 94, same as for the molasses. So we are not going to crunch the full recipe.   Just substitute 232g of honey for the molasses and your macros are the same, 38 30 32. Then, 360g-232g=128g/8=16g, use 16g less per aliquot, 274-16=258g per pour.

	per shake	per batch	per pour
NCD Molasses Shake™	$2.82	360g	274g
NCD Maple Shake™	$3.00	275g	263g
NCD Honey Shake™	$2.81	232g	258g

If you use regular milk instead of raw, the price drops by 75 cents per serving, so closer to $2 per shake. But you miss out on the raw proteins and better probiotics. You won't find this much nutrition anywhere for $3. And with 4.3 grams of Omega-3 freshly ground!

PREVIEW
from the
ABC Water and the Number Crunch Diet

As you know, the recipes for the NCD are being published under the titles, *12 Changes a Year* – the companion guide to the Number Crunch Diet. It may take up to a year to get them written as it will comprise about three volumes. In the meantime, you can get your pH paper testing set up and determine your current alkaline stores. The recipes read like a book and include additional information that I've discovered about diet, lifestyle, health and selfcare. I look forward to seeing you over there!

To join my mission in providing people with safe, effective, affordable, selfcare protocols, send someone you know to www.abcwaterandthenumbercrunchdiet.com. Tell them to take the Quiz!! Thanks for your support! God Bless.

Jumper Publications & Media
From Advice to Results

I almost forgot! (again, not really) to tell you!

If you liked this shake recipe be sure to check out

TCY
12 Changes a Year
Vol 2

for the NCD ORANGE SHAKE!
It makes 9, and I often repeat the recipe midweek.
And whey protein – but not from powder.
And not from cottage cheese either!

BUY THE BOOK!!
IT'S GOOD STUFF!

FREE REPORT #1

JPM Mouth Rinse Protocol™

In the highly competitive world of publishing and creating a following, a reader base, you've always got to give your audience something for free. This way, if the book was not quite what they thought it was worth, the "free" item will hopefully make up for it. Keep in mind, I price things according to what I would pay for them and according to other things. People pay $250 to see a sporting event, but squawk about the price of information that can positively affect their health for decades to come. A one-night stay in your average hotel room while on vacation can cost $179, and it's long gone. Someone told me he sold a used fishing lure on eBay for $400. What's really going to help you on your journey?

As a lifetime seeker of self-improvement, I have never thought twice about the price if I knew it would benefit me. I left Timothy Ferris, author of *The Four Hour Body*, a 5-star review, even though I had to read all 572 pages of his book to get two things out of it. But, it's two things that I didn't have before I read the book. A person with a lot of these Gold Nuggets is miles ahead in the game of life than someone who just goes along never seeking information. So, there's your good advice. And if you are curious to know what those two things are that I got from his book, stay tuned!

Okay, I'll tell you.

This may not be new to some of you but it was to me.
1. Glut Ham Raises – totally works the backs of your legs.

Not just the hamstrings but the calves and butt as well. Attempt to do 12-15 slow reps in 60 seconds and you will feel it the next day. Best bang for your Back-Of-The-Leg buck. However, for erectors, inner hip muscles, I still like single leg "rocking" deadlifts.

2. MED – Minimal Effective Dose
It's best explained like this. Water comes to a boil when it reaches 100 degrees celsius. Adding more heat, more energy, doesn't make it boil more. Applying this to exercise, it's the old "Stimulate Don't Annihilate" rule. Do one set to failure and that's it. Stop. You're done. Let your muscles break down and regrow bigger. It works. And the best part is, you keep cortisol levels under control. Heavy workouts can zap your body for days, especially when you're over 50!

So this is why *ABC Water and the Number Crunch Diet* is priced like a BMW. It's Revelation Information. A synergy of dozens of books and specialties, to create a completely new book. Selfcare.

So your free report is about "How To Improve Your Gums And Teeth". Two words. Hydrogen Peroxide.

But not so fast. There's the detail.

JPM Mouth Rinse Protocol™

I have to give credit to my brother for this one. He is 62, has never had a cavity, and 33-years ago his dentist told him that he doesn't need to keep coming to the dentist, that, "You're your own dentist."

Now, how many people do you know of that have been told by their dentist that their personal dental hygiene is so good that they are their own dentist and that the dentist actually tells them to stop coming to the dentist? I only know of one. My brother. And he has fantastic teeth and gums, and he's 62, retirement age. What was his secret weapon all these years. Hydrogen Peroxide.

I recall a coworker telling me she had so many dental problems and she was so upset about them. I told her to rinse with hydrogen peroxide. She came back the next week with a big smile on her face, all that anxiety that she had was gone, and she sincerely thanked me profusely. She was smiling bigger and I could tell her gums were looking better already.

Lack of Attached Gingiva. Nobody wants to hear their dentist or dental hygienist say this. Gingiva just means gums. Lack of attached gums, means you have pockets. You know, like when they do the probing of your gums, 334 333 233 432. They go around your teeth checking the pockets of your gums at three locations on each tooth, cheek side and tongue side. Bleeding and pockets means GINGIVITIS. Gum Disease. Bad News.

But there's hope. You can, in my experience, and obviously in my brother's experience, have healthy gums by rinsing with hydrogen peroxide. But there's some do's and don'ts, so keep reading.

I will give you the whole protocol that I do so that you can set it up for yourself at home and begin today to drop those pocket measurements from four and three millimeters to two and one millimeters, and yes, it is possible to have zero mm pockets. Zero mm pockets means you have 100% fully-attached gums to your teeth. My brother has this. You can tell when he smiles. He's got solid gums that are gripped solidly on to his teeth. No pockets. No recession. No Lack of Attached Gingiva.

Of course we have all asked him where he got the idea to rinse with hydrogen peroxide. His answer is brilliant.

"I just thought, well, I'll rinse with hydrogen peroxide."

You see, you don't have to be a doctor to know things, or a PhD, or a licensed blah blah blah. My brother is none of those things. Yet he's a genius when it comes to oral hygiene. AND, the most notable part of his discovery is, It Just Came To Him. Like a thought. Or a revelation. He already had a million-dollar smile, so he was thinking about how he could maintain it and improve on it

51

so that he could have that million dollar big teeth square jaw smile for his whole life.

Imagine having perfect teeth and gums and you haven't been to the dentist in 33 years. In the ABC NCD book I talk about not paying too much attention to crossover double-blind placebo-controlled scientific studies. For some things, the obvious answer is right in front of your face. Just look and believe it. I don't need a study to prove to me that hydrogen-peroxide rinsing can transform bad gum tissue into healthy gum tissue and reduce pocket depth. I use it and it does it. Every one of our family members uses it. We are all following my brother's oral hygiene protocol.

So, here's what you do.

Initial Setup. Buy 8 bottles of 15oz Lea & Perrins Worcestershire sauce at the supermarket. Transfer the liquid to a one-gallon container, or discard it, then proceed to thoroughly rinse the bottles and scrub off the labels. Now you have eight 15oz glass amber bottles with tight-fitting screw caps. The amber color will prevent light from degrading the H_2O_2 into water, and the screw cap will prevent oxygen from getting inside and reacting with the H_2O_2 and converting it into water. So your hydrogen peroxide will stay potent. Also, if you haven't already read my website, we here at JPM and ABC NCD are Plastiphobes. We avoid plastics for eating and for anything that will go in our mouth or used on our body. The HUGE one is, never microwave food in a plastic container, and the lesser evils are, storing the shampoo you use on your head in a plastic container. Replace the plastic containers in your kitchen and bathroom with glass wherever possible.

So, this 15oz bottle is ideal and you'll see why as we go along.

Next. Buy a gallon of hydrogen peroxide. I get mine at Smart & Final supermarket and restaurant-supply store, $8. It's the most economical, $1 per 16oz. And a gallon will keep you from running out. Fill your eight worcester bottles full to the top, to the brim, and then cap them. The bottle holds 16oz exactly, so you have the exact amount needed to fill all 8 bottles to the top. If the bottles were really only 15oz, then 8x15=120oz, and a gallon is 128oz, so you would have 8oz left over. BUT, lucky for you, I have already figured out the perfect bottle.

The other reason for using this bottle is because it has a small mouth. You want to be able to control the amount of hydrogen peroxide entering your mouth as you take a "swig". A wide-mouth bottle will have you pouring in too much H_2O_2 into your mouth. This is important because:

1. Hydrogen peroxide is for external use only. Don't Drink it.
2. If you get too much in your mouth, and it makes contact with the back of your throat, your throat will dry out and you'll end up with a raspy voice.

That brings us to the Technique.
Pucker your lips and use your tongue to control the liquid as it enters your mouth. When you have about a tablespoon of hydrogen peroxide in your mouth, half an ounce, close your lips and use your cheeks to swirl the liquid around your teeth and gums.

DON'T LET IT TOUCH THE BACK OF YOUR MOUTH

You will have a raspy voice and dry throat if you do.

H_2O_2 IS NOT FOR GARGLING

I will tell you what to use for oral gargling at the end. Your Second Free Report!

So with the H_2O_2 in your mouth, swirl for 30 seconds minimum or 60 seconds maximum. Any less than 30s and you're not doing it long enough for cleaning action to occur, and any longer than 60s and it's no longer doing anything because it's all deactivated, reacted.

Until you get comfortable with this technique, keep your chin down. The natural reaction is to gargle as you are swirling. Don't.

KEEP YOUR CHIN DOWN in the beginning. After a month, the habit should be solidified and you will be able to keep your head in its natural upright position and multitask or stare at yourself in the mirror as you swirl. Are you looking HYA??

Place one of your worcester 16oz hydrogen-peroxide bottles in the shower for your morning oral-hygiene routine, and place the other in the medicine cabinet above your bathroom sink for your before-bed oral-hygiene routine.

16oz will last about one month, 1T, or half an ounce, times 30 days. So, once a month you will start a new bottle in the shower and a new bottle in the medicine cabinet. This is why eight bottles and the one gallon of hydrogen peroxide is the way to do it. When you run out, you just grab another bottle. Two bottles a month means that your eight bottles will last you four months. So every 4 months, or 16 weeks, 3 times a year, you have to pick up a gallon of H_2O_2 and aliquot it into your eight bottles. This is your system.

I gave a bottle to a friend and he freaked out because his gums were foaming up. I said, "Yeah, your gums are foaming up because your gum lines are dirty." He did it twice a day and on the third day they just foamed up a small normal amount. He thanked me profusely.

And I do mean profusely. People are amazed at how amazing this works for reversing bad gums and for making them look that healthy pink color. And no more sensitive areas after a while.

And I've NEVER heard this anywhere. I honestly believe that when this goes viral, mainstream, because of its effectiveness, that the originator was my brother, back in the 1970s, when something, God maybe, inner Divine Intelligence maybe, said, "I think I'll try rinsing with hydrogen peroxide."

You heard it here first. But the credit goes to my brother Ken!

FREE REPORT #2

JPM Mouth Wash Protocol™

This next one, I will take credit for. And that's the mouth rinse for gargling, aka, mouth wash.

You know, I've never liked using mouthwash. Whenever I tried it, you know, the typical brand they advertise on TV that starts with the letter L, my eyes would get red and my mouth would burn and I'd spit it out and ask myself.

"Why does mouthwash have to feel so toxic?"

Well, fast-forward to the modern world and we now know that IT IS TOXIC. It's loaded with toxic cancer causing birth defect inducing hormone disrupting CHEMICALS!

You will never convince me that thymol, eucalyptol, methyl salicylate, menthol, alcohol, benzoic acid, poloxamer 407, and caramel, are safe and essential for oral hygiene. Salicylate is aspirin. Why does mouthwash need aspirin? To calm the inflammatory effect from all the chemicals.

And that "alcohol", well, it doesn't say if it's ethanol, the drinkable one, but it could be isopropyl alcohol, rubbing alcohol, the poisonous one, or it could be a mixture of the two. Dr. Hulda Clark in her book, *The Cure For All Diseases*, states that she detects isopropyl alcohol contamination everywhere in our lives because the food industry uses it to sanitize. So the next morning they start up the food-processing machines and all that isopropyl alcohol residue ends up in the food. In trace amounts and randomly, yes, but when you are getting exposed to it from every angle, it begins to build up in the body. She stated in her book that every single cancer patient is toxic with isopropyl alcohol.

There's a group of people who bash her books, and I am not saying she was 100% spot-on with every word she wrote, no person is, and she often said when interviewed that, "We haven't discovered that part yet." But her 604-page book is packed with information and it's the reason that today you hear about pollutants, contamination, chemicals, toxins, detox, and purity. I highlighted and underlined more than half of the book and it took me six months to read it.

So although I take credit for this mouthwash, I really need to give credit to the late Dr. Hulda Clark and *The Cure For All Diseases*. You see, vodka is food-grade alcohol. It's the only food-grade alcohol. And alcohol is a good germ-killer, sanitizer, cleaner, and antiseptic.

JPM Mouth Wash Protocol™

Buy a 1.75 liter bottle of vodka, 40% alcohol by volume, not 25%.

I used to buy the Heritage brand 1.75L 40% vodka at Albertson's supermarket for $9.99, $8.99 on sale, plus tax, but the bottle is plastic.

Plastiphobe

So now I buy the "UV" brand 40% vodka in the 1.75L glass bottle. It's $16.99 at Albertson's, but other grocery stores stock it as well.

I spent a while deciding which glass bottle of vodka to go with, and the UV brand won, as the glass is clear, the shape is smooth, and it has indentations at the back for your hand to grip it. Nice.

40% is too strong for gargling so you will want to dilute it 50/50 half-and-half with water. Go to the healthfood store and buy a few bottles of bottled water in glass. Drink the water and remove the labels. I use Voss brand 400mL cylindrical glass water bottles with screw caps. Nice and classy looking when you get the label cleaned off. Place the bottle on your scale and turn it on. Add 200 grams of vodka, then add 200 grams of water. Voila, 20% vodka.

This is your mouthwash for gargling.

As with the worcester bottles, buy eight Voss water bottles so that you have some ready-to-use when you run out. I use this 20% alcohol to rinse my mouth after meals during the day, along with flossing and brushing. For toothpaste I use Trader Joe's/Tom's brand, with Fennel, Propolis and Myrrh, lavender color on the box.

Tom's brand has been around for a long time and back in the 1980s is was the only Health Food toothpaste. In the 1990s they used to put the PURPOSE for their ingredients on the toothpaste box. So, they had a list of about six ingredients in one column, and the purpose for each ingredient right across from it in another column. They stopped doing this. Now they just list the ingredients, and shockingly, GLUTAMATE is ingredient number seven. This is why I don't use toothpaste that frequently. Glutamate, Excitotoxin, is in my Health Food toothpaste. Terrible.

JPM Oral Hygiene AM Protocol™
Brush – toothpaste
Floss
Mouth Rinse – 1T H_2O_2 30-60sec
Mouth Wash – 20% vodka gargle & rinse 10-15sec

Throughout the day and after eating:
Brush – no toothpaste
Floss
Mouth Wash – 20% alcohol gargle and rinse

JPM Oral Hygiene BB Protocol™
Before Bed same as AM

Hard/Firm toothbrush if my tongue feels a gritty film anywhere. Scaling tool once a week on anterior lowers (minerals in my saliva tend to precipitate on the backs of my lower teeth). And I use one of those long Oral B-60 toothbrushes to clean my tongue AM and PM. A lot of people neglect their tongue hygiene.

If you don't already own one, a Must-Have is an electric toothbrush. Hand brushing simply can't compare to the fast vibrating movement of an electric toothbrush. Philips Sonicare $35, works great. I keep one in my car. (No that's not weird.)

I am not as fortunate as my brother in that I still go to get my teeth cleaned every 6-12 months, but my hygienist and dentist always remark at how good my gums look, and how clean my teeth are. Apparently, a lot of teenagers have poor gum health and oral hygiene. Soft drinks! It's liquid sugar. The NCD considers soda pops as poisons, especially acidic colas. They're Anti-Nutrition. Health destroying.

Recall from the ABC NCD that – No amount of good can counter the bad you expose yourself to daily. You've got to eliminate the bad. In the old days, I can remember coke being used to remove the corroded-metal buildup from the posts of a car battery. And it worked good. Think about what it's doing to your teeth and gums.

As a final note, my next project is to discontinue using 3% topical hydrogen peroxide from the body-care aisle, and order 35% food-grade hydrogen peroxide from www.purehealthdiscounts.net. Then, just dilute it to about 3% by adding 1.5 ounces of the 35% H_2O_2 to the worcester bottle and then filling it to the top with water. See *Nontoxic Teeth Whitening and Dental Hygiene System*

And as another word of caution regarding the use of hydrogen peroxide as a mouth rinse.

IT'S NOT RECOMMENDED IF YOU HAVE METAL FILLINGS.

The H_2O_2 will, on a small scale, dissolve the metal, and those metal atoms can then be absorbed into your bloodstream via the capillary beds underneath your tongue, causing you to auto-intoxicate yourself over time. But if you have metal fillings in your mouth, your saliva is doing the same thing to a lesser degree 24-hours-a-day 7-days-a-week. If it was me, I would still do the hydrogen-peroxide mouth rinse AM and PM, as the benefits of having attached gingiva and healthy gums outweighs the risk of trace amounts of metal dissolving, getting into the bloodstream, and traveling to various locations within the body. Best advice is to have them removed and redone with composite, PLASTIC!

As a benefit to using the H_2O_2 mouth rinse AM and PM, you'll have nice white teeth! Peroxide is the active ingredient in most teeth whiteners.

Hope You Enjoyed This.

Jumper Publications & Media
Your First Choice for Selfcare

Once you've set up these two oral hygiene protocols and begin to see the benefits for yourself, why not hit the website and purchase a copy for a friend or family member, boss, coworker or your employees. For $30 you could purchase 10 copies and hand them out as "thank-you" tokens to people you know. Remember, it's fully copyrighted ISBN 978-1502489142 so making copies and free distribution is illegal – and bad Karma!

Leave a Review

Without giving away the contents, "spoilers", recommend this publication and leave a review so that someone else might benefit from it too. Thank you.

www.amazon.com   Search: flaxseed shake recipe

Subscribe to my YouTube Channel
www.youtube.com   Search: Number Crunch Diet

Be sure to send me an email so I can periodically keep in touch with updates and new Selfcare Strategies – and discount offers on new items (yes, more than books!) (a simple and effective weight-loss device) (a weightlifting "device" that I use EVERY time I work out) and don't forget the recipes! – TCY.

abcwaterandthenumbercrunchdiet@mail.com
Privacy – your email address will not be used for anything other than by Jumper Publications and Media.

FOLLOW-UP

You know, I've never liked the idea of brushing with baking soda because I've had in my mind all these years a picture of my dad brushing his teeth with the white-and-blue box of Arm & Hammer baking soda, and I assumed it was the one from the cleaning products aisle, which has contaminants and is too abrasive.

So, that glutamate in my toothpaste, and the fact that something in me, my Divine Intelligence, is telling me it's not good, has led me to rethink the baking soda for brushing.

Well, here's what you do. Buy baking soda in the BAKING aisle at a good-quality supermarket, I buy mine at Trader Joe's Market and it's USP, United States Pharmacopeia grade, the highest grade you can buy. To a 16oz glass jar, add the entire contents of the baking soda, use it to brush your teeth. Just wet the bristles and touch the powder, brush for two minutes, works great. Just the right amount of abrasion, not too rough not too mild. The food-grade USP baking soda in the baking aisle is so finely ground it's like a light soft powder, Perfect. The baking soda also gives your body a slight amount of bicarbonate, sodium bicarbonate, for alkalinity. See *ABC Water and the Number Crunch Diet* for the significance of alkalinity to good health, energy, and being ailment free.

So the JPM Oral Hygiene Protocol™ becomes,

1. food-grade or USP-grade baking soda to brush
2. 3% topical or food-grade hydrogen peroxide for gum lines
3. 20% food-grade vodka to gargle

The hydrogen peroxide and the baking soda will whiten.

If you do buy the 35% hydrogen peroxide, dilute it to 6% instead of 3% for a super-powerful teeth whitener! However, if you just be consistent and do the hydrogen-peroxide mouth rinse protocol AM and PM every day, you won't need more whitener. The 3% twice a day works perfectly. Happy Hygiene!

Saliva vs Urine pH

Top Ten Reasons Why Saliva pH Is Worthless When Compared To Urine pH For Acid-Base Analysis

#10 Small Volume – small tiny volume samples don't represent the whole

#9 Difficult to Obtain – the procedure is to bring up saliva and swallow, 2x, then use the third one for the test, too hard to obtain

#8 Poor Reproducibility – when you retest your saliva sample, you will likely get a slightly different color (reading)

#7 Poor Accuracy – if you collect a second sample, it will likely give you a different reading than the first

#6 Bacterial Contamination – bacteria from your mouth will interfere with the test

#5 Food Contamination – food from your mouth will interfere with the test

#4 Spoon Contamination – the surface of the spoon that you collect it on is going to affect your small sample

#3 Viscosity – saliva is too thick and results in faded or dual colors of the test pad (or paper)

#2 Difficulty Reading – the color doesn't "lock in" so you can take a reading, it tends to change shades through a range

#1 Your Salivary Glands have ZERO to do with Acid-Base regulation. Try Kidneys.

Your kidneys are running your body's alkaline status.

And your alkaline status is the secret they don't want you to know.

JPM Oral Hygiene Protocol

This publication is the introduction to JPM. If you paid $2.99 for the kindle version or $4.99 for the paperback version, then you basically paid for the two protocols, the 20% vodka mouthwash, and the Secret Weapon, H_2O_2 gum-line cleaner. You will notice advertising for the other publications. Don't be upset. You got your $3-5 worth. The same cost as for a venti mocha latte, that's long since gone. The information in this publication will be with you for you to use for the rest of your life, every day.

So, why not take the ABC NCD Quiz!

The first half of the book is all about alkalinity. The secret aspect to your health no one, but a few, will talk about. However, no one covers the subject better and more comprehensively than in ABC Water™. The second half is the Number Crunch Diet™. No recipes, but lots of good sound information on diet. You will learn a lot, as no one discusses it the way I do. I brag a bit about the book, because it's really a great book. It's a compilation of nearly 100 books that I've read. But more of a Synergy, a new approach.

The recipes can be found in *12 Changes A Year* and you can see a sample on www.abcwaterandthenumbercrunchdiet.com

The title *Nontoxic Teeth Whitening and Dental Hygiene System* begins with the two chapters you just read, but includes a one-of-a-kind food-grade teeth whitening system, if you feel you need more whitening. It also includes a commentary on fluoride. Wouldn't you like to know if fluoride's something you should be doing, or something you shouldn't be doing?

So put your thinking cap on and let's start the Quiz!

It's good for you!

Pick the correct answers – There may be more than one

1. A urine pH of 5 is telling you
   a. about your blood pressure
   b. that you're tired
   c. about your alkaline reserves
   d. to see a doctor
   e. that you're healthy and fine

2. Urine pH testing is routinely performed by licensed
   a. social workers
   b. clinical laboratory scientists
   c. respiratory therapists
   d. fitness advisors
   e. nurses and doctors

3. The cost of one month of urine pH testing is _____ the cost of
   open heart surgery (CABG).
   a. 1/10
   b. 1/100
   c. 1/1000
   d. 1/10,000
   e. 1/100,000

4. The opposite of metabolic acid is dietary
   a. phosphates – found in meats and cola drinks
   b. bicarbonate – found in packaged foods
   c. caffeine – found in green tea
   d. bicarbonate – found in fruits and vegetables
   e. bicarbonate – found in oils and fats

5. Information can be of which types
   a. true
   b. incomplete

c. false
d. clouded
e. secret

6. "Natural Flavor" on a food label is
   a. natural flavor extracts from plants and fruit
   b. glutamates, MSG, altered salts
   c. chemicals that make you addicted to the product
   d. generally safe and good for me
   e. not something I need to worry about

7. During World War II, the people who failed to act early
   a. suffered
   b. died
   c. lost everything
   d. became victims
   e. made it through unscathed

8. Compensating means
   a. saving for retirement
   b. eating foods that lift your mood
   c. doing something to mask something
   d. brushing it out of your thoughts
   e. pleasing others and being a do-gooder
   f. all of the above

9. The reason(s) people are fat
   a. they're born that way
   b. they don't make their own meals
   c. hereditary – handed down from your parents
   d. my body just won't lose fat
   e. they don't see the numbers in what they're eating

10. The "Cheat Day" is
   a. a great way to get food cravings satisfied
   b. required to reset my fat-burning hormones
   c. a 2-8 step backwards day
   d. works well for most people long term
   e. is a popular "trick" that you should buy into

ANSWERS

1. A urine pH of 5 is telling you
   a. about your blood pressure – No, but there is a relationship (see Chapter 24)
   b. that you're tired – No, but there is a relationship (see Chapter 20)
   c. about your alkaline reserves – YES! Get to know your alkaline status by reading this book.
   d. to see a doctor – No, but it can lead to that.
   e. that you're healthy and fine – One number tells you little, 35 numbers a week tells you a lot. Get to know your urine pH.

2. Urine pH testing is routinely performed by licensed
   a. social workers – no
   b. clinical laboratory scientists – Yes, 99% of all urine testing is done by a CLS.
   c. respiratory therapists – no
   d. fitness advisors – no
   e. nurses and doctors – Doctors do perform urine tests in their offices, but they are not looking at urine pH with much depth.

3. The cost of one month of urine pH testing is _____ the cost of open heart surgery (CABG)(a bypass, "cabbage").
   a. 1/10 – no
   b. 1/100 – no
   c. 1/1000 – no
   d. 1/10,000 – Yes. You can test all of your urinations for about

$1 a month (see Chapter 11). A cabbage would run you at least $10,000.
  e. 1/100,000 – no. But I believe the potential to save yourself $100,000 in medical treatments is very possible.

4. The opposite of metabolic acid is dietary
  a. phosphates – no, phosphates contribute to acidity
  b. bicarbonate – no, bicarbonate yes, but not from packaged foods
  c. caffeine – no, caffeine is a drug, most drugs are acidic
  d. bicarbonate found in fruits and vegetables – Yes!
  e. bicarbonate found in oils and fats – no, oils and fats are not sources of bicarbonate

5. Information can be of which types
  a. true – Yes, this is a bit what your life is all about. Finding the truth about things.
  b. incomplete – aka, partial truths or half truths, aka, "spin". Do you find your head spinning when you go for fancy medical treatments?
  c. false – lies, yes lies. Don't call them untruths. Lies are Lies. When people lie it's your job to call them on it. Otherwise, "ya got no backbone".
  d. clouded – blurry, muddied, confusion. I could write "scientifically" but I would just make you confused and half lost. How does that help you.
  e. secret – Now we're talking. When they say "buy this stock" you've got to be a moron to buy it. The payoffs and the winners are kept secret, shared through word of mouth.

6. "Natural Flavor" on a food label is
  a. natural flavor extracts from plants and fruit – Well, they would like you to think that, but that's far from reality.
  b. glutamates, MSG, altered salts – Yes, often this is the case.
  c. chemicals that make you addicted to the product – Yes

Absolutely
d. generally safe and good for me – don't buy that line
e. not something I need to worry about – you make your own choices in life

7. During World War II, the people that failed to act early
Referring to this is grim and bleak. But there are people suffering and dying every day because they failed to act early. You could say that WWII is still happening all around us in the United States of America today. My book can help you not to fall victim to this death and suffering. So that you make it through your life, unscathed.

8. Compensating means
a. saving for retirement – no, but I have seen people who are just a little too attached to their portfolios, compensating?
b. eating foods that lift your mood – no, but food is commonly used to compensate
c. doing something to mask something – Ah-Ha, Yes.
d. brushing it out of your thoughts – no. It's okay and healthy to let go of thoughts, just be sure you're not avoiding your issues.
e. people pleasing – reward seekers may be compensating
f. all of the above – no, just C. Go back and read C again.

9. The reason(s) people are fat
a. they're born that way – don't give me that
b. they don't make their own meals – Bingo! This is key.
c. heredity – your fat jeans are because of your fat genes – no I don't think so
d. my body just won't lose fat – I hear you. There is not a lot of good help out there. Luckily, you've found the right place.
e. they don't see the numbers in what they're eating – Yes. And person D above just needs to look at food mathematically (and read the book).

10. The "Cheat Day" is
   a. a great way to get food cravings satisfied – Wrong. I'm a testimony of getting rid of food cravings. See Chapter 38, 39, 40, 41.
   b. required to reset my fat-burning hormones – Wrong. If you get your macros right, your hormones will cooperate just fine.
   c. a 2-8 step backwards day – On page 84 of *The Four Hour Body* the person states that he gains 4.4 lbs on his cheat day. Then he loses it. Can you say "moody"?
   d. works well for most people long term – After reading dozens of diet books, I could not find one that worked long term, so I made my own. It's called the Number Crunch Diet.
   e. a popular "trick" that you should buy into – The Number Crunch Diet isn't about cheating. Although it's full of useful "tricks" that I came up with and use daily.

You'll be miles ahead of the average person after a while.